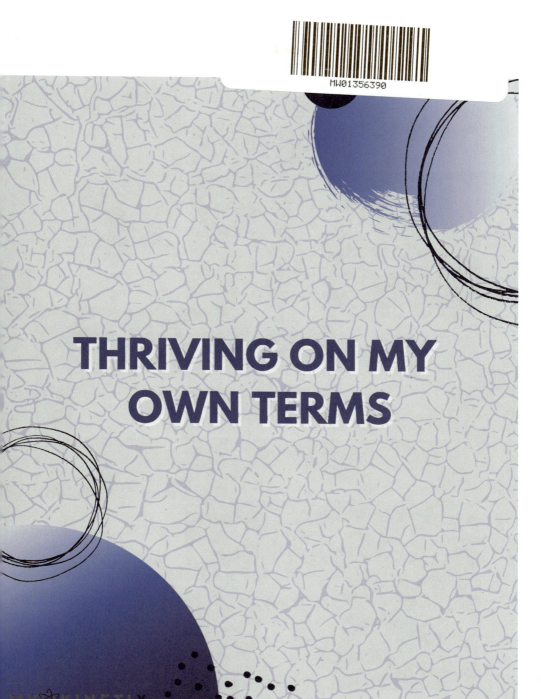

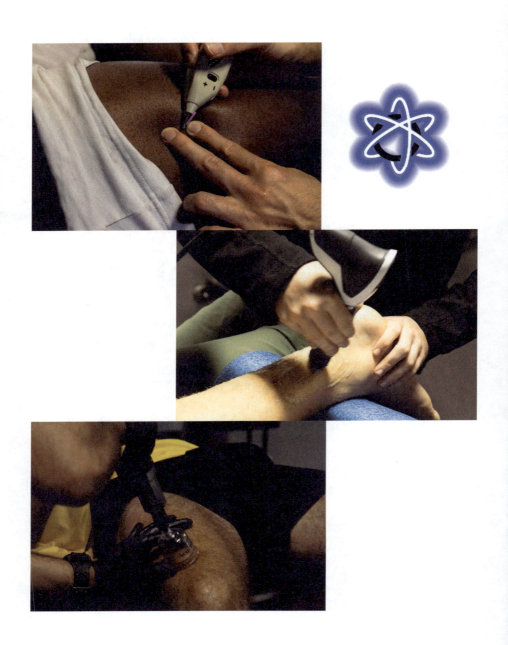

WHAT WE OFFER AND YOUR PROGRESS

OUR SERVICES

Physical Therapy

Acupuncture

Dry Needling

Shockwave Therapy

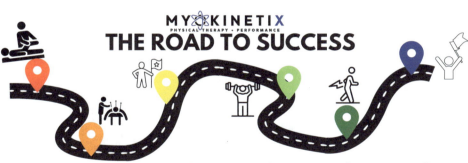

THE ROAD TO SUCCESS

1. EVALUATION
The evaluation stage is all about **YOU**! We do the detective work to find the root cause of your problems.

2. RECOVER
The recover stage involves hands-on care at our physical therapy clinic. The goal of this stage is to address and get rid of your pain.

3. REBUILD
The rebuild stage involves strengthening exercises for the middle stages of your recovery. The goal of this stage is to rebuild your foundation and get back to your baseline.

4. STRENGTHENING
While strengthening, we not only want to get you beyond the baseline of your injury, but in all forms, to prepare you for return to sport or everyday activities.

5. REDEFINE
The goal is to redefine yourself after injury. We want to get you back to the journey you were on before you were injured, which may involve your sports-related drills.

6. THRIVE
This is where you get the ability to fully return to your sport or everyday activities. Relive your life as if the injury didn't occur in the first place, while still coming in to maintain the progress you've made.

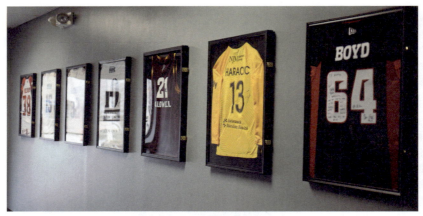

OUR STORY

LIFE IS A SPORT.
EVERYONE IS AN ATHLETE.

It's time to treat your body like an athlete by maximizing your human performance & optimizing your recovery with our PT, acupuncture, & other non-surgical treatments!

Everyone is an athlete to some degree & needs to be treated like one! We are here to help you prepare for whatever life throws at you!

Our doctors of physical therapy strive to care for & improve every individual's needs, movements, & performance while living a healthy & active lifestyle. By solving pain, movement management, & injury prevention we can eliminate the need for numerous doctor's visits or addictive prescription medications. I couldn't have built this alone.

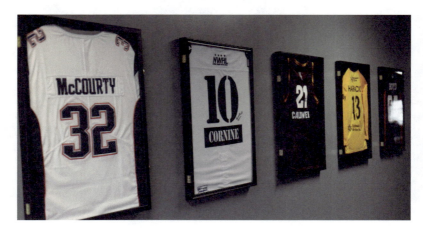

OUR TEAM

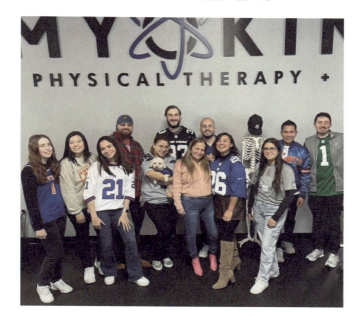

Our team is committed to helping you through your recovery journey!

Scan to learn more!

OUR TRIBE

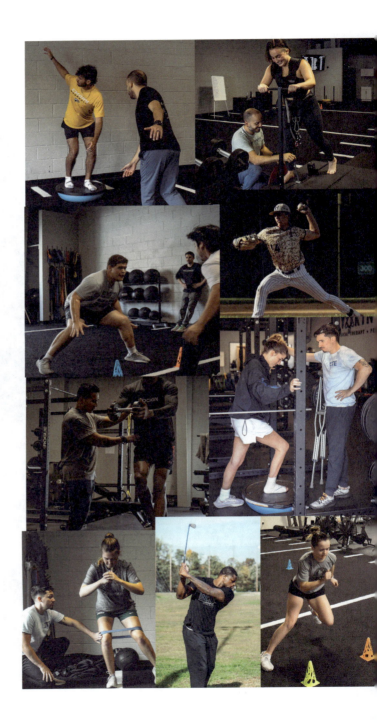

Colleges & Teams Whose Athletes Attended Myokinetix

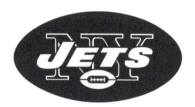
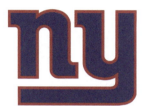
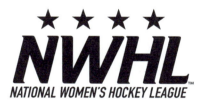
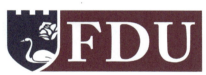
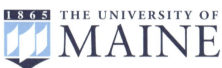
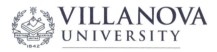
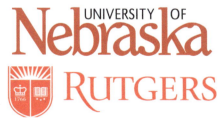
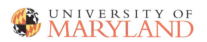
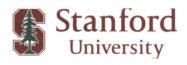
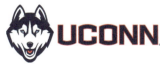

WAGNER COLLEGE

CEO & FOUNDER
DR. NATTY BANDASAK

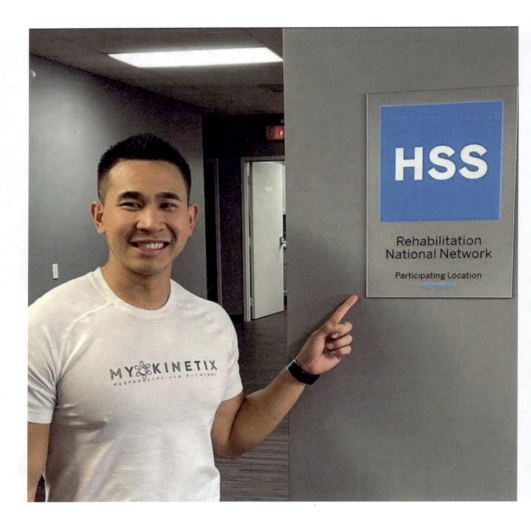

"It all started in 2012 when I severely injured my back working out; I couldn't walk for 2 weeks. I kept wishing that the pain would stop so I could go back to working out & doing what I was passionate about. This started my journey in the Physical Therapy world. After I finished PT, I took the experience with me & applied to Physical Therapy school with the hope of helping people who are going through the same struggle that I experienced.

Fast-forward to 2016 when I received my Doctorate in Physical Therapy & began my career. I was filled with excitement & eager to help as many people as possible. The PT clinic that I worked at was extremely busy & was treating 3-4 patients per hour. I was not able to give the care that my patients deserved due to time restriction. This was when I realized that the healthcare system is broken & was no longer about the patients but rather the profit.

I envisioned a place where patients are being put FIRST & treated like VIPs the first minute they set foot in the door. This was the spark that ignited **Myokinetix Therapy & Performance**.

2018 was the year where I pursued my vision & started a patient-eccentric practice. This was the only way for me to fulfill my true passion for helping people to take their lives back."

SUPPLEMENTS

Myokinetix is proud to be affiliated with Thorne Supplements. Thorne is an NSF Certified manufacturing facility with the most extensive line of NSF Certified for Sport® nutritional supplement products on the market.

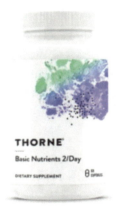 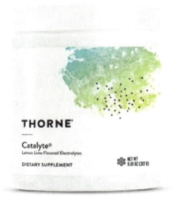 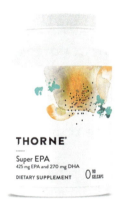

OUR CORE VALUES

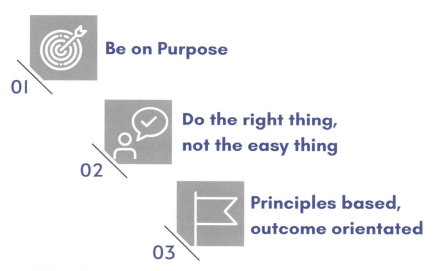

01 — Be on Purpose

02 — Do the right thing, not the easy thing

03 — Principles based, outcome orientated

WE LOVE TO WORK WITH PEOPLE JUST LIKE YOU

Scan QR code to send someone our way!

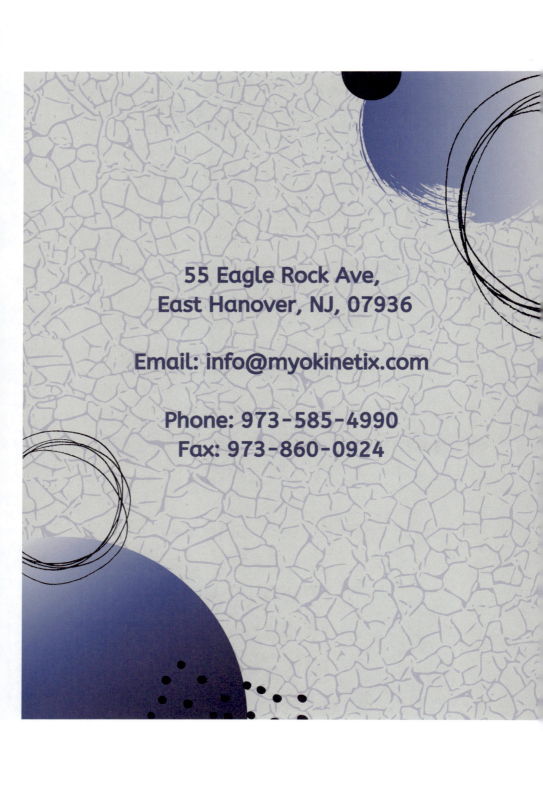

Daily Gratitude Log

DATE:

TODAY I AM GRATEFUL FOR...

TODAY SOMETHING THAT BROUGHT ME JOY IS...

TODAY I AM PROUD OF MYSELF FOR...

TODAY I AM LOOKING FORWARD TO...

If you want to find happiness, find gratitude.

—

STEVE MARABOLI

Things That Bring You Joy

Use this page to make a list of things that bring you joy in life. Write anything that comes to mind. It doesn't matter how small or big it is.

1.
2.
3.
4.
5.
6.
7.
8.
9.
10.
11.
12.
13.
14.
15.

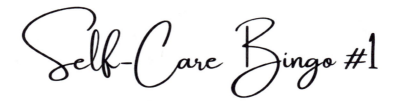

Complete self-care activities to complete the bingo board!

Do a digital detox	Create a morning routine	Help someone in need	Go camping	Learn how to knit
Listen to an motivational podcast	Choose a healthier food alternative	Take a break to stretch	Take a bubble bath	Visit a national park
Go on a hike	Play a board game	SELF CARE	Say no to something	Create something with your hands
Take your vitamins	Go for a walk	Spend some time painting	Go to the dentist	Prioritize your sleep
Try a new hobby	Give yourself a day of rest	Volunteer for a cause you care about	Do something unplanned	Get some fresh air

The more regularly and the more deeply you meditate, the sooner you will find yourself acting always from a center of peace.

—

KRIYANANDA

Things You Have Learned

Use this page to make a list of lessons you have learned in life.

1.

2.

3.

4.

5.

6.

7.

8.

9.

10.

11.

Self-Care Checklist

Create a list of self-care tasks that you would like to complete this week. Use the boxes to check off the days when you completed the tasks.

TASKS	S	M	T	W	T	F	S
	☐	☐	☐	☐	☐	☐	☐
	☐	☐	☐	☐	☐	☐	☐
	☐	☐	☐	☐	☐	☐	☐
	☐	☐	☐	☐	☐	☐	☐
	☐	☐	☐	☐	☐	☐	☐
	☐	☐	☐	☐	☐	☐	☐
	☐	☐	☐	☐	☐	☐	☐
	☐	☐	☐	☐	☐	☐	☐
	☐	☐	☐	☐	☐	☐	☐
	☐	☐	☐	☐	☐	☐	☐
	☐	☐	☐	☐	☐	☐	☐

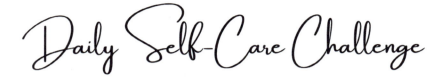

Daily Self-Care Challenge

DAY 1:

Pick a moment during the day when you are feeling stressed and take a 10-minute break to do a quick stretch routine. Stand up and stretch your arms above your head, reach for your toes, roll your shoulders, and stretch your neck from side to side. Repeat each stretch a few times, breathing deeply and focusing on the sensation in your body.

DAY 2:

Start your day with a healthy breakfast. Choose foods that give you energy and nourishment, such as whole-grain toast, fruit, or yogurt. Take a moment to appreciate the flavors and textures of your food, and savor each bite.

DAY 3:

Disconnect from technology for an hour today. Turn off your phone, computer, and other devices, and spend time doing something that doesn't require screens, such as reading, writing, or drawing. Notice how it feels to be fully present in the moment, without distractions.

DAY 4:

Get some fresh air and exercise. Take a walk or jog outside, or do some yoga or stretching in a nearby park. Notice the sights, sounds, and smells of nature, and let yourself feel invigorated by the movement and activity.

DAY 5:

Take a relaxing bath or shower. Light candles, play calming music, and use your favorite soaps, shampoos, and lotions. Let yourself unwind and release any tension or stress from your body.

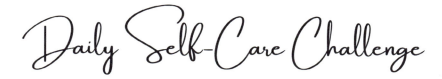

Daily Self-Care Challenge

DAY 6:

Make time for a hobby or creative pursuit. Whether it's painting, writing, or gardening, spend some time doing something that brings you joy and fulfillment. Let yourself be fully immersed in the activity, without worrying about the outcome or results.

DAY 7:

Take a few minutes today to reflect on the things in your life that you're thankful for, whether it's a supportive friend, a cozy home, or a good cup of coffee. Write down three things that you're grateful for, and carry that sense of appreciation with you throughout the day.

DAY 8:

Connect with a friend or loved one today, especially one you haven't spoken with in a while. It can be through a phone call, text, or video chat. Social connections are important for our well-being.

DAY 9:

Take a few minutes today to practice deep breathing or meditation. Even a few minutes of meditation can help reduce stress and anxiety, and promote relaxation.

DAY 10:

Treat yourself to something you enjoy, whether it's your favorite food, a movie, or a hobby you haven't had time for lately.

Positive Quotes

Use this page to write down your favorite positive quotes. They can be about self-care, having gratitude, mindfulness, etc. We started the list for you!

"Self-care is not selfish. You cannot serve from an empty vessel." - Eleanor Brown

"Acknowledging the good that you already have in your life is the foundation for all abundance." - Eckhart Tolle

Self-Care Bingo #2

Complete self-care activities to complete the bingo board!

Practice self-compassion	Do something nice for someone else	Go for a run	Learn a new gym exercise	Cook yourself a healthy meal
Practice deep breathing	Spend some time at a beach or lake	Schedule your annual physical	Take a break from social media	Share your feelings with a loved one
Spend time in nature	Go for a swim	**SELF CARE**	Organize one area of your house	Offer support to a friend
Watch your favorite TV show	Listen to an audiobook	Forgive yourself for a mistake	Say yes to something new	Practice yoga
Learn how to set boundaries	Check on your mental health	Give yourself a massage	Treat yourself to a snack	Spend some time gardening

Things You've Accomplished

Sometimes in life we are scared to do certain things or feel like we aren't capable enough to achieve them. Use this page to make a list of things that you have accomplished in your life.

1.
2.
3.
4.
5.
6.
7.
8.
9.
10.

Things To Let Go Of

Use this page to make a list of things that you would like to let go of. These could be such as negative thoughts, past mistakes, unhealthy relationships, or even physical clutter in your home.

1.
2.
3.
4.
5.
6.
7.
8.
9.
10.

Positive Affirmations

I am capable of achieving anything I set my mind to.

I am grateful for all the opportunities and blessings in my life.

I am surrounded by love and support.

I am confident in my abilities and skills.

I am strong and resilient, and I can overcome any obstacle.

I am proud of my accomplishments and my progress.

I am worthy of love and respect.

I am at peace with myself and my life.

I am constantly learning and growing and embracing change.

I trust that everything will work out for my highest good.

The goal of meditation isn't to control your thoughts, it's to stop letting them control you.

—

UNKNOWN

My Favorite Books

Use this page to make a list of books that you enjoyed reading. You can use this list as a reference when you are looking for good books to read again or recommend to others.

TITLE: AUTHOR:	TITLE: AUTHOR:
TITLE: AUTHOR:	TITLE: AUTHOR:
TITLE: AUTHOR:	TITLE: AUTHOR:
TITLE: AUTHOR:	TITLE: AUTHOR:
TITLE: AUTHOR:	TITLE: AUTHOR:

Books to Read

Use this page to make a list of books you would like to read!

1.
2.
3.
4.
5.
6.
7.
8.
9.
10.
11.

My Reading Journal

TITLE:

AUTHOR:

WHAT WAS YOUR FAVORITE PART OF THIS BOOK? WHY DID IT RESONATE WITH YOU?
_____
_____
_____
_____

HOW DID THIS BOOK MAKE YOU FEEL? WHY DO YOU THINK YOU FELT THAT WAY?
_____
_____
_____
_____

WHAT IS SOMETHING THAT YOU LEARNED FROM THIS BOOK?
_____
_____
_____
_____

DID THIS BOOK INSPIRE YOU IN ANY WAY TO MAKE CHANGES IN YOUR LIFE?
_____
_____
_____
_____

WOULD YOU RECOMMEND THIS BOOK TO OTHERS?   YES   NO

People Who Inspire You

NAME OF PERSON:

WHY DOES THIS PERSON INSPIRE YOU?

WHAT QUALITIES OF THIS PERSON WOULD YOU LIKE TO ATTAIN?

NAME OF PERSON:

WHY DOES THIS PERSON INSPIRE YOU?

WHAT QUALITIES OF THIS PERSON WOULD YOU LIKE TO ATTAIN?

Things You Are Thankful For

Use this page to make a list of things you are thankful for in life. Think about your relationships, your health, your living situation, yourself, etc.

1.
2.
3.
4.
5.
6.
7.
8.
9.
10.
11.

When You're Feeling Down...

Practice self-compassion

Reach out to someone

Engage in physical activity

Practice mindfulness

Do something you enjoy

Engage in acts of kindness

Get some fresh air

Practice good self-care

Practice gratitude

Seek help if needed

Self-Care Techniques

PRACTICE SELF-COMPASSION

Be kind to yourself and acknowledge that it's okay to feel down sometimes. Treat yourself with the same empathy and understanding you would offer to a friend in a similar situation.

PRACTICE MINDFULNESS

Engage in mindfulness techniques, such as deep breathing, meditation, or body scans. These practices can help you become more present and calm your mind.

ENGAGE IN PHYSICAL ACTIVITY

Physical activity can release endorphins, which are known as "feel-good" hormones. Take a walk, go for a run, do some yoga, or engage in any form of exercise that you enjoy.

ENGAGE IN ACTS OF KINDNESS

Doing something kind for others, whether it's volunteering, helping a friend, or performing a random act of kindness, can boost your mood and sense of purpose.

Self-Care Techniques

DO SOMETHING YOU ENJOY

Engage in activities that bring you joy, such as reading a book, watching a movie, listening to music, cooking a meal, or engaging in a hobby. Doing things you love can help shift your focus and lift your mood.

GO OUTSIDE

Spending time outdoors, whether it's going for a walk in nature, sitting in a park, or simply opening a window, can help you feel refreshed and rejuvenated.

TAKE CARE OF YOUR BODY

Take care of your physical health by getting enough sleep, eating nourishing foods, and staying hydrated. Taking care of your body can positively impact your mood and well-being.

PRACTICE GRATITUDE

Reflect on the things in your life that you are grateful for, whether it's big or small. This can help shift your focus from negativity to positivity.

Gratitude Meditation

Gratitude meditation is a powerful practice that can help shift your focus to the positive aspects of your life and cultivate a sense of appreciation.

Find a quiet and comfortable place to sit or lie down. Close your eyes and take a few deep breaths, allowing your body and mind to relax.

Bring your attention to the present moment and begin to reflect on the things in your life that you are grateful for. Let go of any distractions or negative thoughts, and allow yourself to fully immerse in the feeling of gratitude.

QUESTIONS TO ASK YOURSELF:
- What are you grateful for about your body?
- What are you grateful for about your immediate environment?
- Who are you grateful for and why?
- What are you grateful for about your life experiences?
- What are some qualities or values you have that you are grateful for?

Take a few more deep breaths, and when you're ready, gently open your eyes. Take a moment to savor the feeling of gratitude and carry it with you as you go about your day.

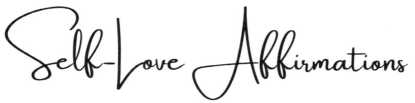

Write down 10 things that you love about yourself.

1.

2.

3.

4.

5.

6.

7.

8.

9.

10.

Acknowledging the good that you already have in your life is the foundation for all abundance.

—

ECKHART TOLLE

My Favorite Foods

Write down your top 10 favorite foods!

1.
2.
3.
4.
5.
6.
7.
8.
9.
10.

My Favorite Desserts

Write down your top 10 favorite desserts!

1.
2.
3.
4.
5.
6.
7.
8.
9.
10.

My Favorite Recipe

Think of a meal or snack that brings you joy even when you are feeling down. Save the recipe for it below!

INGREDIENTS:

DIRECTIONS:

NOTES:

Self-Care Bingo #3

Complete self-care activities to complete the bingo board!

Go on a road trip	Learn how to play an instrument	Spend time with animals	Make a calming playlist	Spend some time dancing to relax your body
Write a thank you note	Draw a self-portrait	Celebrate something accomplished	Daily journal for a week	Speak kindly to yourself
Go stargazing	Practice meditation for 15 min	SELF CARE	Stick to a bedtime routine	Go on a nature walk
Call a loved one	Stay hydrated	Watch your favorite movie	Practice mindfulness	Learn how to bake a new treat
Prioritize your well-being	Give yourself words of affirmation	Spend 30 minutes reading	Express your feelings through writing	Do something nice for yourself

Gratitude makes sense of our past, brings peace for today, and creates a vision for tomorrow.

—

MELODY BEATTIE

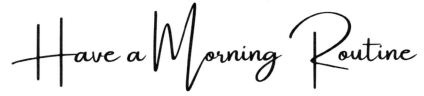
Have a Morning Routine

The key to a morning routine is to create one that works best for you. Make it something that you can do daily. Starting your day with intention and self-care can set the tone for a positive and productive day ahead!

WAKE UP EARLY
Start your day by waking up at a time that allows you to complete your morning routine without feeling rushed. Choose to wake up at the same time each day.

HYDRATE YOUR BODY
Drink a glass of water as soon as you wake up to rehydrate your body after a night of sleep and kickstart your metabolism.

EXERCISE / DO YOGA
Spend a few minutes stretching or doing some light exercises to wake up your body and get your blood flowing.

PRACTICE MEDITATION
Take a few moments to center your mind and set a positive tone for the day ahead.

PREPARE FOR THE DAY
Take a few moments to review your schedule for the day, set goals or intentions, and plan out your tasks and priorities. This can help you feel more organized and focused as you go about your day.

Create Your Morning Routine

The key to a morning routine is to create one that works best for you. Make it something that you can do daily. Starting your day with intention and self-care can set the tone for a positive and productive day ahead!

TIME	TASK

Things You Are Proud Of

Use this page to make a list of things that you are proud of yourself for doing. These may be things that you accomplished that you originally were afraid to do or thought you couldn't do.

1.
2.
3.
4.
5.
6.
7.
8.
9.
10.

Reframing Negative Thoughts

Use this page to work through any negative thoughts that you are having.

IDENTIFY NEGATIVE THOUGHTS
Thinking about yourself and your life, write down any negative thoughts that come to mind. Write freely without judging or filtering anything that comes up.

QUESTION THE THOUGHTS
For each negative thought identified above, ask yourself whether there is any evidence to support it. Reflect on other possibilities or explanations for the situation causing the negative thought.

REFRAME THE THOUGHTS
After reflecting on each negative thought, try to convert it into a positive thought. Think about what you really know about the situation and find something positive about it to focus on instead.

Workout Routine

Design your workout routine to match your fitness goals and lifestyle. Try to set achievable goals that you can meet every week.

MONDAY

TUESDAY

WEDNESDAY

THURSDAY

FRIDAY

SATURDAY

SUNDAY

Simple Exercises

Try one of these simple exercises everyday to get yourself moving. Daily activity is important because it helps maintain physical health, improves mental well-being, and reduces the risk of chronic diseases.

JUMPING JACKS

Stand with your feet together and jump, spreading your legs and raising your arms overhead. Jump back to the starting position and repeat.

PUSH-UPS

Start in a plank position with your hands shoulder-width apart and your body in a straight line. Lower your body until your chest almost touches the floor, then push back up.

SQUATS

Stand with your feet shoulder-width apart and squat down, keeping your back straight and your knees over your toes. Stand back up and repeat.

LUNGES

Step forward with one foot and lower your body until your front knee is at a 90-degree angle. Return to the starting position and repeat with the other leg.

The greatest wealth is health.

———

VIRGIL

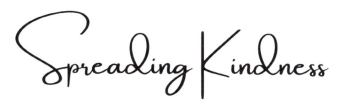

Spreading Kindness

- Give a thoughtful compliment
- Smile and say hello to someone new
- Volunteer your time for a cause you care about
- Send a care package to a friend or family member
- Have patience with someone during a difficult situation
- Leave a positive review for a small business
- Hold the door open for someone
- Reach out to a friend to check in
- Help someone with a task they are struggling with
- Surprise a loved one with their favorite food or activity

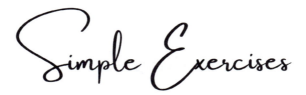

Simple Exercises

Try one of these simple exercises everyday to get yourself moving. Daily activity is important because it helps maintain physical health, improves mental well-being, and reduces the risk of chronic diseases.

PLANK

Start in a push-up position, but instead of lowering yourself to the ground, hold your body straight from head to heels.

BURPEES

Start in a standing position, then squat down and place your hands on the ground. Jump your feet back into a plank position, do a push-up, jump your feet back to your hands, and then jump up back to a standing position.

BICYCLE CRUNCHES

Lie on your back with your hands behind your head and your knees bent. Lift your head, shoulders, and feet off the ground and pedal your legs in the air as if you were riding a bicycle.

MOUNTAIN CLIMBERS

Start in a plank position, then bring one knee up toward your chest and then back to the starting position. Repeat with the other knee.

Simple Exercises

Try one of these simple exercises everyday to get yourself moving. Daily activity is important because it helps maintain physical health, improves mental well-being, and reduces the risk of chronic diseases.

JUMP ROPE

Start by holding one end of the rope in each hand in front of you, then swing the rope over your head behind you and back around in front of you with the rope passing under your feet on the way. Jump over the rope as it passes under your feet.

WALL SIT

Stand with your back against a wall and your feet shoulder-width apart. Lower yourself down into a squat position and hold for as long as you can.

HIGH KNEES

Stand with your feet hip-width apart and run in place, lifting your knees up to hip height with each step.

MOUNTAIN CLIMBERS

Start in a plank position, then bring one knee up toward your chest and then back to the starting position. Repeat with the other knee.

Meditation is a way for nourishing and blossoming the divinity within you.

—

AMIT RAY

Self-care is not selfish.
You cannot serve from
an empty vessel.

—

ELEANOR BROWN

Movies to Watch

Use this page to make a list of movies you want to watch!

1.
2.
3.
4.
5.
6.
7.
8.
9.
10.
11.

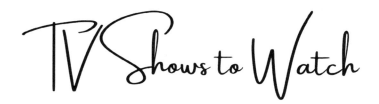

Use this page to make a list of TV shows you want to watch!

1.
2.
3.
4.
5.
6.
7.
8.
9.
10.
11.

Gratitude Journal

DATE:

TODAY I AM GRATEFUL FOR...

TODAY SOMETHING THAT BROUGHT ME JOY IS...

TODAY I AM PROUD OF MYSELF FOR...

TODAY I AM LOOKING FORWARD TO...

Gratitude Meditation

Take a few minutes at the end of the day to write down three things that you are grateful for that happened during the day. Try to be as specific as possible and think about how each of these things made you feel.

DATE:

1.

2.

3.

After you've written down your three things, read each one again and allow yourself to feel the gratitude and appreciation for each of them. By focusing on the positive happenings in your life, you will naturally start to feel more fulfilled and attract more positive things into your life.

When I started counting my blessings, my whole life turned around.

—

WILLIE NELSON

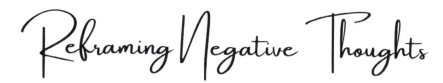

Reframing Negative Thoughts

STEP 1: IDENTIFY A NEGATIVE THOUGHT

Thinking about yourself and your life, write down any negative thought that come to mind. Write it down freely without judging or filtering.

STEP 2: QUESTION THE THOUGHT

Ask yourself whether there is any evidence to support the negative thought identified above. Reflect on other possibilities or explanations for the situation causing the negative thought.

STEP 3: REFRAME THE THOUGHT

After reflecting on the facts related to your negative thought, you will likely find that what you are thinking is not the only possibility or explanation. Convert your negative thought into one or more positive thoughts by choosing to focus on positive explanations for your situation.

Nourishing yourself in a way that helps you blossom in the direction you want to go is attainable, and you are worth the effort.

―

DEBORAH DAY

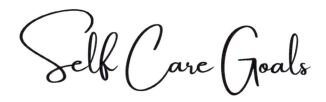

MENTAL HEALTH GOALS:

1.

2.

3.

PHYSICAL HEALTH GOALS:

1.

2.

3.

PERSONAL GROWTH GOALS:

1.

2.

3.

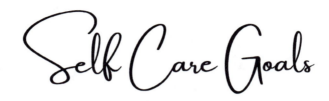

CAREER GOALS:

1.
2.
3.

FINANCE GOALS:

1.
2.
3.

ORGANIZATION GOALS:

1.
2.
3.

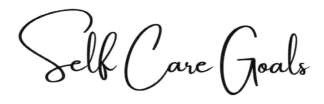

Self Care Goals

FRIENDSHIP GOALS:

1.

2.

3.

FAMILY GOALS:

1.

2.

3.

RELATIONSHIP GOALS:

1.

2.

3.

Daily Planner

DATE:

TO DO

NOTES

IMPORTANT EVENTS

:	AM / PM	
:	AM / PM	
:	AM / PM	
:	AM / PM	

Daily Planner

DATE:

TO DO

NOTES

IMPORTANT EVENTS

:	AM / PM	
:	AM / PM	
:	AM / PM	
:	AM / PM	

Weekly Planner

WEEK OF:

MONDAY

TUESDAY

WEDNESDAY

THURSDAY

FRIDAY

SATURDAY

SUNDAY

Monthly Goals

MENTAL	PHYSICAL	SELF-GROWTH

CAREER	FINANCE	ORGANIZATION

FAMILY	FRIENDSHIPS	ROMANCE

Yearly Goals

MENTAL	PHYSICAL	SELF-GROWTH

CAREER	FINANCE	ORGANIZATION

FAMILY	FRIENDSHIPS	ROMANCE

Self-Care Assessment 1

I prioritize my physical well-being by engaging in regular exercise and maintaining a healthy lifestyle.

STRONGLY DISAGREE — SLIGHTLY DISAGREE — NEUTRAL — SLIGHTLY AGREE — STRONGLY AGREE

I allocate time for activities or hobbies that bring me joy and relaxation.

STRONGLY DISAGREE — SLIGHTLY DISAGREE — NEUTRAL — SLIGHTLY AGREE — STRONGLY AGREE

I make sure to get enough sleep and prioritize a consistent sleep schedule.

STRONGLY DISAGREE — SLIGHTLY DISAGREE — NEUTRAL — SLIGHTLY AGREE — STRONGLY AGREE

I regularly practice stress management techniques, such as deep breathing, meditation, or mindfulness.

STRONGLY DISAGREE — SLIGHTLY DISAGREE — NEUTRAL — SLIGHTLY AGREE — STRONGLY AGREE

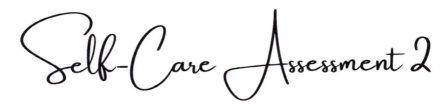

Self-Care Assessment 2

I establish healthy boundaries and say no when I need to, without feeling guilty.

| STRONGLY DISAGREE | SLIGHTLY DISAGREE | NEUTRAL | SLIGHTLY AGREE | STRONGLY AGREE |

I make time for social connections and nurture supportive relationships with family and friends.

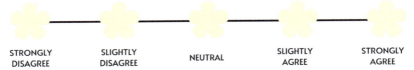

| STRONGLY DISAGREE | SLIGHTLY DISAGREE | NEUTRAL | SLIGHTLY AGREE | STRONGLY AGREE |

I listen to my body's needs and take breaks when necessary to rest and recharge.

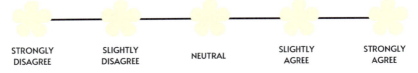

| STRONGLY DISAGREE | SLIGHTLY DISAGREE | NEUTRAL | SLIGHTLY AGREE | STRONGLY AGREE |

I prioritize self-compassion and practice positive self-talk to promote a healthy self-image.

| STRONGLY DISAGREE | SLIGHTLY DISAGREE | NEUTRAL | SLIGHTLY AGREE | STRONGLY AGREE |

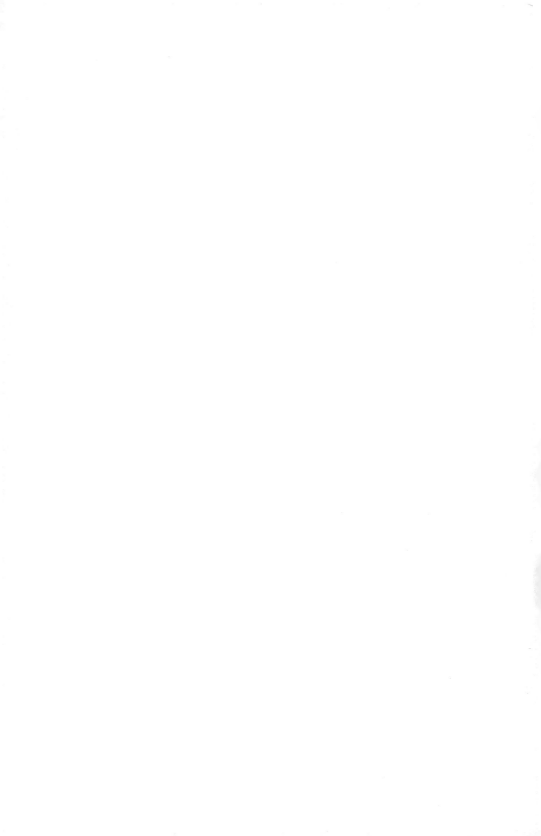

Made in the USA
Columbia, SC
30 January 2025